EFFECTIVE ANSWERS
To Your
WEIGHT LOSS QUESTIONS

Sabinah Oroge

TABLE OF CONTENTS

INTRODUCTION

How many diets plans have you tried over the years? Have you ever stopped dieting because the plan you were on did not work for you? Have you ever wondered why? What diet plans are there - have you heard of any or all of these ones?

- 5:2 diet
- Dukan diet
- Paleo (or paleolithic) diet
- Atkins diet
- Alkaline diet
- Cambridge diet
- South Beach diet
- Jenny Craig diet
- Paleo Diet
- Slimming World diet
- Slim-Fast diet
- Lighter Life diet
- Weight Watchers diet
- Rosemary Conley diet
- The Harcombe diet
- The DASH diet
- The TLC diet
- Mediterranean diet
- Raw Food diet

Have you heard of many of the latest ideas? Would you prefer not to have to count calories when you diet? What about high-protein, high-fat and low-carbohydrates as a diet? Do you know the difference between low-fat and low-carbohydrate foods? And why is some fat in your food good for you?

And why does sugar appear in so many foods nowadays? Not just in soda but also peanut butter! In fact, are low-fat processed meals good for you at all? And what about "cheat days" and "binge eating" - why are they harmful to your diet? Can you drink wine or beer when you diet? Can you lose weight if you always eat out? You will be surprised at what we suggest.

And how many calories do you need to eat a day in order to lose weight? What is your Body Mass Index (BMI) and what should you do about it? How often should you weigh yourself? The answers to these questions may surprise you.

All of these questions, and more, are answered in this book. You will find helpful advice in the answers to assist you in losing weight. There is even a five-day diet plan, based on the Harcombe diet, to give you a kick start. We even give advice on what to do when you reach your goal weight.

In case you are wondering, we have spent a LONG time researching the answers shown here to 25 or so of the common questions asked about weight loss through dieting. The information supplied is based on the latest current medical understanding of how our bodies absorb the foods we eat and what strategies we should follow if we want to shed unwanted weight.

We do not recommend any particular diet plan, because the choice is yours. You need to be happy about what you are eating, and you need to learn about portion-size control for yourself.

And exercise is strongly recommended – not just because turning fat into muscle makes you look thinner, although that is a good thing (muscle has greater density than fat, so 1 kilo of muscle is smaller than 1 kilo of fat). We cannot recommend an exercise plan for you as it depends upon what you want to do. You do not need to go to a gym or get a personal trainer, though. You can jog around your local park, take up cycling, and go swimming regularly. Just be active.

It is easy to measure weight, just jump on the bathroom scales, but what about fat? Fat around the thighs or buttocks seems to be less of a health risk to that on the waist. The recommendation is to have a waist-size (measured at the tummy button) equivalent to less than half you height. Whilst losing weight, you want to retain as much muscle as you can. One of the questions describes metabolism and the importance of keeping your muscle bulk as you age. It is a real aid to weight loss.

So stop reading this section and get straight on to the questions and their answers. You will not be disappointed.

YOUR QUESTIONS ANSWERED

1. Do I have to exercise or just stick to dieting alone?

We often hear that a little exercise is a key to weight loss. For example, use the stairs instead of taking an elevator. But research shows that it is better to cut down our calorie intake. To achieve a 300 calories energy deficit, you can run in the park for 3 miles, or not eat 2 ounces of potato crisps (or chips). Studies that compare exercise with dieting show that participants tend to lose weight by dieting alone than by exercise alone. Both together are even better as they work in harmony.

Exercise has effects on hunger and appetite hormones. These make you feel noticeably hungrier after exercise. If you walk briskly for an hour and burn 400 calories, and then have a slice of pizza with some beer as the exercise made you hungry, you will eat more calories than you burned off. It may not be pizza with beer, but people do often naturally compensate for calories burned.

For every action there is a reaction, we learn in physics, but this law seems to work in biology too. Our body has compensatory mechanisms to counteract the effect of exercise. When we exercise a lot and get tired, we may well rest for the remainder of the day. Some of the calories we burn come from our normal movements during the day. So if you become tired after exercise and then sit on the couch for the rest of the day, you may well lose the energy deficit gained from the exercise.

2. To lose weight, how many calories do I have to burn?

You need to expend more calories per day than you eat, for your body to lose weight.

Your body has a base metabolic rate (BMR), which equates to a set number of calories a day. If you eat more calories than your body needs, you will gain weight. Many studies have found that in general women need 1,500-2,000 kcal to maintain their current weight and for men the range goes to 2,000-2,500 Kcal. In essence this figure gives you the number of calories your body needs on a daily basis in order to function properly. This is not how many calories you consume per day, but how many calories your body needs to function.

If you consistently eat fewer calories than your body needs in a day, it will start to convert body fat into energy to keep going. If you starve yourself long enough, your body will start using its own muscle fibre as an energy source. Remember that you use energy to digest food. So you have to be balanced about thinking of calories alone.

Remember that 1 pound of fat = 3,500 calories approximately. This means that if you consume 3,500 more calories than what you burn in a period of time you will gain one pound in weight. But if you manage to burn 3,500 more calories than you consume you will lose 1 pound in weight.

So to lose weight, you need to eat fewer calories than your body needs to run itself, OR increase your BMR by exercising more. But be careful... Not eating enough during the day slows down your metabolism two ways. First, your body thinks it's starving, so it will slow down your calorie-burning capacity in order to "survive." Second, you are likely to make up for low-caloric intake in the last few hours of the day, causing your body to hang on to the food through the night in preparation for another day of "starving."

3. Explain the use of the BMI calculator?

The Body Mass Index (or BMI) is a way of seeing if your weight is appropriate for your height. The actual calculation is your weight (in pounds) divided by your height (in inches). BMI is divided into several categories, and generally the higher your

BMI, the greater your risk of a large range of medical problems. The chart below indicates the weight in pounds and height in feet and inches. For example if an individual is 5 feet 10 inches and weighs 140 pounds; the BMI is 20.1 which is considered normal. On the other hand, if the same individual weighs 190 pounds, the BMI is 27.1 and the person is referred to as being overweight while a BMI of 34.4 for the same individual (with a weight of 240 pounds) is considered obese. If the same individual has a weight of 120 pounds, the BMI is 17.2 and the person is said to be underweight. You can easily determine your BMI if you know your weight and height.

Weight in Pounds

Height	100	110	120	130	140	150	160	170	180	190	200	210	220	230	240	250
4'	30.5	33.6	36.6	39.7	42.7	45.8	48.8	51.9	54.9	58.0	61.0	64.1	67.1	70.2	73.2	76.3
4'2"	28.1	30.9	33.7	36.6	39.4	42.2	45.0	47.8	50.6	53.4	56.2	59.1	61.9	64.7	67.5	70.3
4'4"	26.0	28.6	31.2	33.8	36.4	39.0	41.6	44.2	46.8	49.4	52.0	54.6	57.2	59.8	62.4	65.0
4'6"	24.1	26.5	28.9	31.3	33.8	36.2	38.6	41.0	43.4	45.8	48.2	50.6	53.0	55.4	57.9	60.3
4'8"	22.4	24.7	26.9	29.1	31.4	33.6	35.9	38.1	40.4	42.6	44.8	47.1	49.3	51.6	53.8	56.0
4'10"	20.9	23.0	25.1	27.2	29.3	31.3	33.4	35.5	37.6	39.7	41.8	43.9	46.0	48.1	50.2	52.2
5'	19.5	21.5	23.4	25.4	27.3	29.3	31.2	33.2	35.2	37.1	39.1	41.0	43.0	44.9	46.9	48.8
5'2"	18.3	20.1	21.9	23.8	25.6	27.4	29.3	31.1	32.9	34.7	36.6	38.4	40.2	42.1	43.9	45.7
5'4"	17.2	18.9	20.6	22.3	24.0	25.7	27.5	29.2	30.9	32.6	34.3	36.0	37.8	39.5	41.2	42.9
5'6"	16.1	17.8	19.4	21.0	22.6	24.2	25.8	27.4	29.0	30.7	32.3	33.9	35.5	37.1	38.7	40.3
5'8"	15.2	16.7	18.2	19.8	21.3	22.8	24.3	25.8	27.4	28.9	30.4	31.9	33.4	35.0	36.5	38.0
5'10"	14.3	15.8	17.2	18.7	20.1	21.5	23.0	24.4	25.8	27.3	28.7	30.1	31.6	33.0	34.4	35.9
6'	13.6	14.9	16.3	17.6	19.0	20.3	21.7	23.1	24.4	25.8	27.1	28.5	29.8	31.2	32.5	33.9
6'2"	12.8	14.1	15.4	16.7	18.0	19.3	20.5	21.8	23.1	24.4	25.7	27.0	28.2	29.5	30.8	32.1
6'4"	12.2	13.4	14.6	15.8	17.0	18.3	19.5	20.7	21.9	23.1	24.3	25.6	26.8	28.0	29.2	30.4
6'6"	11.6	12.7	13.9	15.0	16.2	17.3	18.5	19.6	20.8	22.0	23.1	24.3	25.4	26.6	27.7	28.9
6'8"	11.0	12.1	13.2	14.3	15.4	16.5	17.6	18.7	19.8	20.9	22.0	23.1	24.2	25.3	26.4	27.5
6'10"	10.5	11.5	12.5	13.6	14.6	15.7	16.7	17.8	18.8	19.9	20.9	22.0	23.0	24.0	25.1	26.1
7'	10.0	11.0	12.0	13.0	13.9	14.9	15.9	16.9	17.9	18.9	19.9	20.9	21.9	22.9	23.9	24.9

Height in Feet and Inches

http://www.freebmicalculator.net

Underweight   Nomal   Overweight   Obesity

BMI charts are calculated for adults only. There are separate charts available for children's weight and heights. Inaccuracies can occur if you are an athlete or very muscular as this can give you a higher BMI even if you have a healthy level of body fat and the adult BMI chart is not appropriate for women who are pregnant or breastfeeding, or people who are very frail.

As BMI is based on weight and height, by losing weight you will reduce your BMI and put yourself into a lower risk group. A healthy diet, including a balance of food groups, vitamins and minerals, is essential for a long and active life. Keeping it simple, body weight and shape are a balance of energy intake (dietary calorific content) against output (calorific burn from activity & exercise).

4. Is it harder to lose as one gets older? Is this true?

As someone gets older, the body loses some lean muscle mass every year. The rate is about 2-3% per decade. With the loss of muscle, it becomes harder to lose weight, as your metabolism slows down. "Metabolism" is a word for the chemical reactions that occur in your body to keep it alive, conversion of food into energy and building materials.

5. Why does metabolism slow down as one gets older?

Metabolism is a word for the chemical reactions that your body undergoes to keep it alive. The process of metabolism is what allows you to grow and eventually have children. Your body has a basal metabolic rate (BMR) - the rate at which these processes occur. You might have a high BMR (which allows you to lose weight easily) or a low BMR (which makes you gain weight). The BMR is determined by many factors, and the most important ones are your age, your sex, your height, your body weight, and your activity level.

Metabolism is like all chemical processes and slows down as you age. Your BMR slows down due to the loss of lean muscle mass, which makes it difficult for you to lose weight. The decrease may be 2-3% with each decade. In women, oestrogen levels drop after menopause. This drop causes thyroid hormones that regulate metabolism to drop too.

As your BMR slows down, your body burns fewer calories than before, and this can lead to weight gain if you do not cut down your calorie intake as well.

6. Do men lose weight faster than women?

Men and women have many different physical characteristics. Men are usually more muscular than women. Muscles burn more energy than body fat.

Women are predisposed to store and retain fat. Women have higher levels of oestrogen, a hormone that works to keep the fat on a woman's body so it's easier for her to get pregnant. That means women have to work harder to lose weight at the same rate as men.

Men's bodies respond more quickly to exercise. Women's bodies, meanwhile, actually go into a sort of starvation mode, slowing the metabolism to hang onto more fat.

Women may have a lower tolerance for exercise. Women have smaller lung capacity than men, which can make women feel as though they are working harder than men even if the women are working at the same level. This can also make exercise feel harder in high heat or humidity conditions.

7. What can I do about food craving, how can I stop it?

a) **Distractions** – "If only chocolate will do", is a craving, not hunger. Cravings usually last about ten minutes. Recognize that and distract yourself: phone someone, make some tea, listen to music, sing, run an errand, or simply exercise.

b) **Destroy the temptation** – If you have given in and bought a box of chocolates or biscuits, and feel guilty when eating them, destroy them. Pour water or something else over them to make them uneatable. Do not think about the money you are wasting. If the chocolates or biscuits do not go into the rubbish bin, they are going onto your hips or tummy.

c) Be nutty - Drink two glasses of water and eat an ounce of nuts (for example 20 peanuts). Within 20 minutes, this will extinguish your craving and dampen your appetite.

d) Avoid triggers – Change what you eat. The longer you avoid your trigger foods, the less likely you may be, to want them. In fact, you may begin to crave the foods you DO eat on your diet.

e) Reduce your stress levels - Since cravings can be brought about by stress, learning to deal with stress could potentially save you hundreds of calories a day. This takes some effort and may require you to learn some techniques to manage your stress.

f) Avoid or Plan - Vary your usual routine so you don't normally walk past the bakery, or pizza restaurant. If you know you will be face-to-face with some cake at work, build a portion into the day's calories for your diet.

8. If I cut carbohydrates completely from my diet, can it harm me, is it unhealthy?

If you cut carbohydrates out of your diet for a couple of weeks, you will lose weight. It is one of the best ways to lose weight. Without insulin, your body will lose weight very easily. The only foods that make your body produce insulin are carbohydrates – this is why cutting out carbohydrates can have such an amazing effect.

To have maximum impact you probably want to do the first stage of the Atkins diet. This allows for no more than about 20 grams of carbohydrates each day - so this would allow you a small portion of green vegetables or salad with each of your main daily meals and NO other carbohydrates. No pasta, bread, potatoes, coloured vegetables, fruit, rice, etc.

Your body burns carbohydrates for energy. Depriving it of carbohydrates forces it to turn to fat for fuel – which is a state called "**ketosis**". If you follow a very low- or no-carbohydrate diet you might lose more weight than on a low-fat diet since you are eating less overall. Researchers have not yet determined the long-term effects of ketosis on human health. It is possible that this IS a very healthy way of eating, as opposed to cutting, say, all fat from your diet.

9. If I eat at night; can it hurt my weight loss efforts?

When you eat a meal late at night, it does not permit the body to be active enough to burn off the calories you have eaten within a few hours of finishing the meal. Health experts suggest that going to bed soon after eating means that more calories are converted to fat. They suggest you stay up for at least two or three hours after a meal, and one hour after a snack.

Additionally, staying up should mean maintaining some level of activity, not slouching in front of the TV. Sitting in a recliner chair is the same as going into the bed. The recliner is where a lot of people tend to get into trouble, as there is a tendency to relax at the end of the day, and to indulge in snack foods. If you stay up very late, a snack at midnight is fine, as long as you plan it into the overall daily calorie schedule, and that you stay up for long enough to digest it. The best thing is to eat healthy snack, a carrot or a cucumber will do just well.

10. I am on diet, how often should I weigh myself?

It is generally recognised that a weekly weighing is best. Doing it daily can cause "scale obsession" whereby you become obsessed with how much you weigh. With things like water retention, weight can vary by as much as five pounds throughout the day, so it is vital that you weigh yourself at the same time each time you get on the scales to get a meaningful figure. Weighing yourself weekly does not give the same gratification as weighing yourself each day but it does mean you actual progress downwards to your goal weight can be very pleasing. If you start to see that your dieting effort is paying off, it can be very motivating. Without the constant daily nag of the scales, you can have more of a worry-free diet and feel less pressured. You can concentrate on the diet, and be more at ease when you eat. If you have a slip up one day, there is still time to recover before the scales hand down their next judgement.

So weigh yourself at the same time each week, for example, on a Saturday morning, before you eat anything.

11. How effective are supplements for weight loss? Will taking them help my cause?

Are there weight loss supplements that are safe and helpful during a diet? The following is a list of products you can get from some health food or pharmacies that have some weight-loss evidence behind them:

- Green tea extract
- Meal replacements
- Calcium
- Fibre
- Conjugated linoleic acid (CLA)
- Etc.

Please remember to check with your doctor before taking any type of supplement. Supplements can have side effects and may interfere with any medications you take. And, when it comes to weight loss, there are no quick fixes. Only healthy eating and exercise have been proven to result in weight loss.

That is why dieters are recommended to focus on eating low-calorie foods that have bulk like whole fruits and vegetables, in addition to grains and low-fat dairy and meat. Also, start a fitness program and start to move about more - standing more, taking the stairs, or walking. Change your environment, too, so that it is supportive of a healthy lifestyle - keep fresh fruit in your office, plan meals, and take your lunch to work with you.

12. I am trying to lose weight, can I drink alcohol? If yes or no, why?

Alcohol contains what are known as "empty calories". They do not contribute anything worthwhile to your body's need for nutrients. So it is best to cut down or eliminate all alcohol from your diet when trying to lose weight. Use those calories for foods your body REALLY needs.

Drink alone does not cause a "beer belly", but there are links between alcohol and fat metabolism. When you drink alcohol, your liver slows down its conversion of fat and carbohydrates into energy to eliminate the "dangerous" alcohol in your bloodstream first of all.

If you burn more calories than you eat or drink, you will lose weight. And while alcohol on its own will not inhibit weight loss unless you drink too much too often, drinking alcohol can have a negative result on your chances of eating properly, sleeping well and leading a healthy life style.

13. Is it possible for me to lose weight since I do not cook, I eat out all the time?

Yes, you can if you follow these suggestions.

a) **Beware of "light" dishes.** More and more restaurants are promoting low-calorie, healthy choices, but, unfortunately, the claims are not always true. Read the menu carefully. Look for a mix of lean protein (fish, chicken breast, pork tenderloin, strips of steak), complex carbohydrates (brown rice, whole wheat pasta) and mono-unsaturated fats (canola or olive oil). If you need more information to help you choose the healthiest meals, go to the restaurant's website ahead of time to check if they list nutritional information for each dish they serve.

b) **Don't be afraid to ask.** Restaurants will try and meet all kinds of special requests - all you have to do is ask. Ask for your food to be grilled (or baked, broiled, poached, or steamed) instead of fried. Ask for dishes to be cooked with some olive oil instead of butter.

c) **Practice portion control.** Eat three-quarters of what is on your plate and then stop. This simple step can easily shave up to 300 calories off your meal. What is more, you will be satisfied from eating 75 percent of your dinner, and you will barely miss those extra few bites.

d) **Be smart about salad.** At the salad bar, fill your plate with vegetables, greens, chickpeas, and Japanese edamame, and top it with one or two tablespoons of low-fat dressing. Skip the bacon lardons, cheese, bread croutons, and creamy dressings, and the pasta, tuna, or chicken salads swimming in mayonnaise. If you can't resist, restrict yourself to JUST a quarter-cup serving.

e) **Pick the right protein.** So you must have steak? A 10-ounce rib-eye can be 700 calories or more. Instead, order a leaner cut of beef, such as tender-loin, flank steak, or strip. The recommended serving size is approximately 5 ounces (you can measure this as being approximately the size of the palm of your hand). If the restaurant does not offer one that small, cut your portion in half and take the uneaten part home (in a doggy bag).

f) **Make healthy changes.** Choose whole grains such as brown rice or whole-grain bread over refined white rice and bread. Avoid French fries and the cheese-stuffed potato and order two vegetables, steamed, or a salad and vegetables. Instead of pasta dishes with cream, opt for those with tomato sauces, which are generally lower in fat and calories.

g)Be careful with how much wine you drink. If you want a glass, by all means have it. Just do not go overboard. One study found that women who indulged in more than two drinks a day consumed nearly 30 percent more calories. Stick to one glass of wine. A 125g glass of white wine has about 77 calories, red has 85 calories.

h)Eat dessert. This is not a joke. Try to deny yourself the chocolate pudding that sounds so delicious and you just might eat something worse (like an entire tub of ice cream) when you get home. The smart strategy is to order one dessert for the table. A few bites should satisfy your sweet tooth. You don't want to share today? Ask for a dish of berries or a small fruit sorbet.

14. I have been told that protein shakes are good for weight loss, will they bulk me up?

The energy used up in making carbohydrate, for example, available to the body as energy compared to the energy used up converting protein to usable energy is substantially different. 100 calories of carbohydrate eaten may make 93 available to the body; 100 calories of protein eaten may make only 70 available. – See Jequier, "Pathways to Obesity", International Journal of Obesity, (2002).

Most people gain all of the protein they need from eating a normal diet. Protein shakes provide protein in a particularly easy-to-digest way. Weight trainers need extra protein to build muscle when exercising. The main problem with a lot of these protein shakes is that they also have other ingredients such as carbohydrates and artificial chemicals to enhance colour and taste.
Protein shakes will only bulk your body up when you combine them with exercises that build muscle. That is their purpose.

15. Once I reach my ideal weight, can I stop exercising?

Dieting should be seen in two phases, the first phase is to lose your excess weight, and the second phase is to keep the weight off. When you get to your ideal weight, you need to learn how to eat and exercise without changing your weight. So you can increase what you eat gradually, or decrease the amount you exercise gradually, until you reach a weight plateau that you are happy with. You may find that you still need to exercise, but not as much as you were doing during the first dieting phase.

16. If I reduce my eating and still do not lose weight, what should I do?

Increase the amount of calories that your body burns by increasing the amount of exercise you do. Start going for a jog in the morning, walk or bicycle to work instead of using the car or public transport, use stairs instead of the elevator.

Try a high protein high fat, low carbohydrate diet, such as the Harcombe diet, to refresh your weight-loss. The Harcombe diet plan involves keeping your protein and carbohydrate intake separately and retraining your body to use protein for energy instead of the quick energy you get from carbs. You can find out more about it on their website.

17. How many cheat days can I have per week of dieting?

The short answer is NONE. This might sound hash, but here are some reasons.

If you cheat, your body does not adapt to your new healthy diet. When you drastically change the way you eat, a certain adaptation process takes place. For example, if you are doing a low-carb ketogenic diet, then your body needs to change certain hormones and ramp up production of enzymes to make use of fat as the primary source of fuel. If you keep cheating, you will prevent this metabolic adaptation from ever fully completing. Also, when you abandon the standard western diet and start eating more real foods, it can take some time for the sense of taste to adapt. If you have ever done the "paleolithic" diet for an extended period of time without cheating, then you may have experienced this. With time, real foods start to taste much better. If you cheat and eat junk foods frequently, your taste sensations will not adapt completely and you will not be able to experience the same satisfaction from real foods.

You might binge and eat way too much. Some people can binge like there is no tomorrow and ruin a week's worth of dieting in one sitting. It has been known for bingers to eat 5,000 calories in one sitting. That is two days' worth of calories for a grown man and an entire week (or two) of dieting pretty much ruined.

Cheating does not raise metabolism or prevent "starvation mode". The concept of "starvation mode" is largely a myth with no real science behind it and does not really happen until you get to an extremely low body fat percentage. For healthy people trying to stay healthy or lose a bit of weight, cheat meals are unnecessary at best and may be detrimental.

If you are worried about your metabolic rate going down during a weight loss period, lift weights. This is actually proven to maintain both your metabolic rate and your muscle mass.

Those nasty ingredients will never completely leave your body. Trans fats, seed oils and gluten - these nasty ingredients linger in the body for a while and it takes a long time to fully recover from their effects. If you keep eating them, they will never completely leave your body.

18. If I drink a lot of water, can it cause weight gain?

About 70% of your body is water. You need to take in about 2 litres of water a day to stay hydrated. When you get dehydrated, your body starts to suffer. Your thinking ability deteriorates; you will feel increasingly tired with little stamina. Your mouth and eyes will feel dry. Lack of water can even inhibit a person's workout routine.

Being dehydrated can actually cause you to gain weight. Water helps us to maintain a healthy weight by suppressing our appetite, reducing our body's level of sodium and helping us to maintain muscle tone. Dehydration causes a person to become hungrier, resulting in higher calorie consumption throughout the day.

So ensure you stay hydrated. Drink plenty of fluid every day, water, green tea, coffee. Not soda or beer.

19. Can sugar make me to gain weight?

Most western processed food contains sugar to improve the taste. Until recently, nutritionists suggest that people should get only 10% of their calories from sugar, now WHO recommends 5%. Getting 10% equals 13 teaspoons of sugar per day (based on 2,000 calories per day), while 5% equates to 6.5 teaspoons per day! The current average for an American is 42.5 teaspoons of sugar per day!

A 12 oz. can of soda, such as Pepsi or Coca Cola, has the equivalent of 10 teaspoons of sugar in it. How many do you drink each day?

See this breakdown of where else we get sugar in our diet:

Percentage Item
10%   Sweetened fruit drinks
 5%   Candy
 5%   Cake
 4%   Ready-to-eat cereal
 4%   Table sugar and honey
 4%   Cookies (biscuits) and brownies
 4%   Syrups and toppings

26%   Prepared foods such as ketchup, canned vegetables and fruits and peanut butter

Another high-sugar category is **low-fat products**, which may not be as good for your diet as you might believe. Some contain A LOT of sugar to make up for the lack of the fat which often gives food its taste. So the calorie count of the low-fat version of your favourite mayonnaise may not be much different from the full-fat original.

Once you start checking for sugar in the processed foods in the supermarket, you will find it almost everywhere. Sugar is used to add flavour to foods instead of fat. The food industry has done this as a way of getting us to continue to eat what they manufacture.

20. How can I reduce my fat belly?

Increase the amount of time you exercise. Try doing some squats and dead-lifts to strengthen the muscles in your back and stomach area.

Eat healthy food you cook from scratch. Concentrate on these examples:

Proteins: Eat plenty of lean meat, poultry, fish, whey, eggs, cottage cheese.

Vegetables: Spinach, broccoli, salad, kale, cabbage.

Fruits: Banana, orange, apple, pineapple, pears.

Fats: Olive oil, fish oil, real butter, nuts, flax seeds.

Carbs: Cut down on your carb intake. Eat brown rice, oats, whole grain pasta.

Reduce your alcohol intake. To lose your belly fat, what you drink is as important as what you eat. A little alcohol from time to time is OK. But forget about losing your belly fat if you drink beer & "alcopops" daily. Beer drinkers always have a pear shape: belly fat and man boobs – especially as they get older. Alcohol also stresses your liver which has to work hard to clear the toxins from your system. This gets in the way of building muscles.

21. What can I do to boost my metabolism?

As you age you lose about 2-3% of lean muscle tissue per decade. This naturally reduces your metabolism as you get older. To reverse this, you have to work hard to increase your muscle mass by exercising. Take up weight training.

22. Which 5 exercises can I do to lose weight?

a) **Tai Chi.** This is a Chinese martial art that incorporates movement and relaxation, good for both body and mind. It has been called "meditation in motion." Tai chi is made up of a series of movements, one transitioning gracefully into the next. Tai chi is accessible, and valuable, for people of all ages and fitness levels, because classes are offered at various levels.

b) **Swimming**. Swimming is almost the perfect workout. The buoyancy of the water supports your body and takes the strain off painful joints so you can move them more fluidly. Swimming is good for individuals with arthritis because it is less weight bearing. Research finds that swimming can improve your mental state and put you in a better mood. Water aerobics is another option. These classes help you burn calories and tone up.

c) **Strength training.** If you believe that strength training is a macho, brawny activity, think again. Lifting light weights will not bulk up your muscles, but it will keep them strong. Muscle also helps burn calories. The more muscle you have, the more calories you burn, so it is easier to maintain your weight. Strength training might also help preserve your ability to remember.

Before starting a weight training program, be sure to learn the proper way to do it. Start light with just one or two pounds. You should be able to lift the weights 10 times with ease. After a couple of weeks, increase that by a pound or two. If you can easily lift the weights through the entire range of motion more than 12 times, move up to slightly heavier weight.

d) **Walking.** Walking is simple yet powerful. It can help you stay trim, improve cholesterol levels, strengthen bones, keep blood pressure in check, lift your mood and lower your risk for a number of diseases (diabetes and heart disease for example). A number of studies have shown that walking and other physical activities can improve memory and resist age-related memory loss.

All you need is a well-fitting and supportive pair of shoes. Start with walking for about 10-15 minutes at a time. Over time you can start to walk farther and faster until you are walking for 30 to 60 minutes on most days of the week.

e) **Kegel exercises**. These exercises will not help you look better, but they do something just as important - strengthen the pelvic floor muscles that support the bladder. Strong pelvic floor muscles can go a long way toward preventing incontinence (involuntary urination) While many women are familiar with Kegels, these exercises can benefit men too.

To do a Kegel exercise correctly, squeeze and release the muscles you would use to stop urination or prevent you from passing gas. Alternate quick squeezes and releases with longer contractions that you hold for 10 seconds, and the release for 10 seconds. Work up to three 3 sets of 10-15 Kegel exercises each day.

23. Which 5 diet strategies can I use to shed some pounds from my belly?

a) Cut down on the amount of alcohol you drink. Eliminate it totally if possible. Alcoholic drinks contain what are known as "empty calories" and your body has to work hard to get rid of the poison that alcohol is. When it is doing this, it can't digest the food you've eaten to make it work for you.

b) Exercise more. You don't need to visit the gym. You can cycle or walk briskly around town. Visit the swimming pool regularly.

c) Eat healthy food. Avoid processed foods with extra sugar in.

d) Keep hydrated. Drink plenty of water, tea and coffee - at least two litres a day.

e) Manage your stress. When you are stressed, your body chemistry changes. You may find that you become hungry at strange times and your will power to resist snacks will decline. You may be drawn to unhealthy but easily-available foods, such as confectionary. As much as possible, try not to succumb.

24. How can I reduce my flabby arms?

You need to improve the tone of the muscles in your arms. Take up exercise that will strengthen these muscles, such as swimming or tennis. You could try weight training at the gym as well.

25. Can I have meal plans for 5 days from one or two popular diets including breakfast, lunch, dinner and dessert/snacks to help with weight loss?

The following information comes from the Harcombe, Atkins and Paleo Diets web sites.
Harcombe Diet - It is a reduced-calorie kick-start plan. Men should eat a bit more protein.

Day 1
Breakfast: Bacon and eggs.

Lunch: Salmon steak with selection of vegetables (not potatoes or mushrooms) and a large side salad; natural live yoghurt.

Dinner: Brown rice (50g dry weight) and vegetables (not potatoes or mushrooms) stir-fried in olive oil. Have some fresh raspberries and yoghurt for dessert.

Day 2
Breakfast: 100g brown rice cereal (from the gluten-free section in supermarkets) with water (not milk).

Lunch: Salad Niçoise: a tin of tuna or a tuna steak on a bed of salad. Hard-boiled eggs, olives and anchovies are optional. Olive oil and black pepper for dressing.

Dinner: Meat (steak, or pork chops or lamb etc) with any amount of vegetables (not potatoes or mushrooms) and a salad. Have some fruit for dessert with some yoghurt.

Day 3
Breakfast: Plain or ham omelette (ensure the ham contains just ham and water, not added sugar etc.) made with 2-3 eggs, knob of butter, ½tsp herbs, ground black pepper, chopped ham (optional).

Lunch: Chicken and/or beef strips stir-fried in olive oil with vegetables (not potatoes or mushrooms).

Dinner: Stuffed peppers: boil 50g dry weight brown rice, stir-fry chopped mixed vegetables (not potatoes or mushrooms) in olive oil, then mix the rice and vegetables together and fill a deseeded pepper shell. Bake in a medium oven for 20-30 minutes until the pepper is soft to the touch. Eat some strawberries and cream for dessert.

Day 4
Breakfast: Up to 75g porridge oats with water (put the dry oats in a bowl and pour boiling water on top to the consistency you like).

Lunch: Chef's salad: a large mix of salad leaves, grated carrots and beetroot - be really creative, with cold cuts of meat and/or hardboiled eggs. Olive oil and black pepper for dressing.

Dinner: A large whole fish, such as trout or mackerel, with plenty of vegetables (not potatoes or mushrooms) and salad. Have a banana for dessert.

Day 5
Breakfast: Scrambled eggs (no toast) or soft-boiled eggs with raw vegetable crudité 'soldiers'.

Lunch: Roast or grilled chicken and salad and/or vegetables (not potatoes or mushrooms).

Dinner: 50-75g dry weight rice pasta in a tomato sauce: stir-fry an onion and a garlic clove in olive oil, add a tin of tomatoes, 2tsp basil and black pepper. Simmer until the pasta is ready. Have some fruit for dessert with some yoghurt.
Reproduced from the Harcombe Diet website.

Atkins Diet – This is a low carb diet programme aimed at achieving weightloss.

DAY 1
BREAKFAST: Atkins Advantage Morning Bar (3 net carbs), 2 boiled eggs (1)

SNACK: 1/4 cup ricotta (2), 1 celery stalk (1)
LUNCH: Salmon salad: 8oz/225g salmon mixed with 2 tablespoon mayo, 1 tablespoon parsley, 1/2 cup sliced cucumber (1), 2 cups mixed salad leaves (2).

Top with 4 spears asparagus (2) and 2 tablespoon vinaigrette (2)

DINNER: 8oz/225g grilled chicken breast, 1/2 cup roasted broccoli (1), 1 cup cos lettuce, 2oz/ 57g Parmesan (2), five olives (1), Caesar dressing (1)

SNACK: 1/2 cup sugar-free jelly (1), 2 tablespoon cream (1/2)
TOTAL: 20 1/2g

DAY 2
BREAKFAST: Florentine omelette: 2 eggs (1), 2oz/56g grated cheddar (2), 1 cup chopped spinach (1), 3 bacon rashers (1).

SNACK: 1/2 avocado (2)

LUNCH: Chicken salad: 8oz/225g chicken mixed with 1/2 cup sliced cucumber (1), 1/2 cup cherry tomatoes (2), dill, 2 tablespoon mayo, 2 cups mixed leaves (2), vinaigrette (2)

DINNER: 1 cup clear broth (1), sautéed prawns: 8oz/225g prawns, sautéed in butter, garlic (1), chopped parsley, 2 cups cos lettuce (2), 5 black olives (1), creamy ranch dressing (2)

SNACK: 1oz /28g Edam (1)
TOTAL: 22g

DAY 3
BREAKFAST: 1 slice rye toast (3), 2 sliced smoked salmon, 2 tablespoon cream cheese (1)

SNACK: 1 boiled egg (0.5)

LUNCH: 1 cup chicken broth, Chef salad: 2 slices each of thick ham, turkey, roast beef, 1 chopped boiled egg (1), 1oz/28g blue cheese, 2 slices bacon crumbled over three cups mixed salad (3), vinaigrette (2)

DINNER: 8oz/225g grilled steak with 1/2 cup each of courgette and mushrooms, sautéed (2.5), 1 cup rocket (1), 1/2 cup sliced cucumber (1), ranch dressing (1).

SNACK: Hot chocolate: 1/2 cup plain soya milk, 1 tablespoon cocoa, 1 tsp Splenda (3)
TOTAL: 19g

DAY 4
BREAKFAST: 2 scrambled eggs (1), 1 slice rye toast (3), 2 bacon rashers.

SNACK: A stick of celery filled with 2 tablespoon of cream cheese (3).

LUNCH: 8oz/225g turkey burger with 1 tablespoon ketchup (1), 2 cups lettuce (2), 1 oz/28g crumbled feta cheese and vinaigrette (2).

DINNER: 8oz/225g grilled tuna, 1/2 cup steamed artichoke hearts (2), 2 cups mixed salad leaves with vinaigrette (4).

SNACK: Atkins Advantage Chocolate Peanut Butter Bar (2)
TOTAL: 20g

DAY 5
BREAKFAST: Spiced turkey and egg scramble: 3oz/85g turkey mince with 2 scrambled eggs (2). Season with salt, red pepper flakes and hot pepper sauce.

SNACK: 1oz/28g Swiss cheese (1)
LUNCH: Chicken soup: 8oz/ 225g shredded poached chicken, 1/2 cup mushrooms (1 1/2) in 1 cup chicken broth (1), 2 cups endive (1), 5 olives (1), vinaigrette (2).

DINNER: 8oz/225g roasted pork tenderloin, 3 cups cos lettuce (3), 1oz/28g crumbled blue cheese (1), 2 tablespoon sundried tomatoes (2), vinaigrette (2).

SNACK: 1 stalk celery, 2 tablespoon soy nut butter (2)
TOTAL: 19.5g

Reproduced from the Atkins Diet website.

Paleo Diet – The diet samples below contain a balanced amount of Paleo foods. You are at liberty to adjust the menu based on your preferences.

Day 1

- **Breakfast:** Eggs and vegetables, fried in coconut oil. One piece of fruit.

- **Lunch:** Chicken salad, with olive oil. Handful of nuts.

- **Dinner:** Burgers (no bun), fried in butter, with vegetables and some salsa.

Day 2

- **Breakfast:** Bacon and eggs, with a piece of fruit.

- **Lunch:** Leftover burgers from the night before.

- **Dinner:** Salmon, fried in butter, with vegetables.

Day 3

- **Breakfast:** Meat with vegetables (leftovers from night before).

- **Lunch:** Sandwich in a lettuce leaf, with meat and fresh vegetables.

- **Dinner:** Ground beef stir fry, with vegetables. Some berries.

Day 4

- **Breakfast:** Eggs and a fruit.

- **Lunch:** Leftover stir fry from the night before. A handful of nuts.

- **Dinner:** Fried pork, with vegetables.

Day 5

- **Breakfast:** Eggs and vegetables, fried in coconut oil.

- **Lunch:** Chicken salad with olive oil. Handful of nuts.

- **Dinner:** Steak with vegetables and sweet potatoes.

Courtesy of the Authority Nutrition website.

For the Paleo diet, in the beginning, there is usually no need to track calories or macronutrients.

But, if you need to lose a lot of weight, it is advisable to cut down on carbohydrates and limit your intake of nuts and potatoes.

CONCLUSION

If you have read this whole book, you will have read a lot of advice on dieting and exercise. These two things go hand-in-hand when it comes to losing weight. You have to change your whole approach to life to get down to your goal weight, not only change what you eat but be much more active than you might have been before.

It is hoped that at least some of these questions (a compilation from a survey held) were things you have thought about before. Hopefully, the answers you read gave you some information to help you overcome your problem with weight loss.

AND you do not have to count calories to lose weight. You just have to learn to be careful about what you do eat and with the portions of food that you eat. Please remember, with any diet, ensure you eat a variety of foods and consume all the vitamins and minerals you need each day. And make sure you do not eat much salt or sugar each day, either!

As for exercise, it is not intended that you need to get yourself a personal trainer, unless of course you can easily afford to pay for one, much like Hollywood stars seem to do. You do not even need to book into a gym. You can exercise around your home, by walking more, or cycling to the shops, taking the stairs instead of the elevator at the shopping mall or at work. This is not to say that communal exercise in the gym is wrong, in fact that may be what YOU need to keep on exercising.

And when you get to your goal weight, can you stop exercising? What do you need to remember? Go back and check the answer to that question. That is question number 15

If you apply the advice given, try out any or all of the five-day diet plans; exercise more, and cut down on your sugar intake, there is no doubt at all that you will see real weight loss. When you change your weight, you will feel a whole lot better about yourself. You will not fear the scales, the photographer or shopping for new clothes!

So, go for that new you. Start dieting and exercising **TODAY!**

Go from flabby to **FABULOUS!!!**